LOW RESIDUE DIET COOKBOOK

150 Low Residue Recipes for Soothing Digestive Distress and Embracing Wellness with Healthy Smoothies for Perfect Living

EDWARD LINDA

Table of Contents

INTRODUCTION

A low residue diet is meant to put as few demands on the digestive tract as possible. It's similar to a low fiber diet, but it also excludes some foods that can stimulate bowel contractions. "Residue" refers to material left in your digestive tract after the initial stages of digestion are finished. These materials often contain a lot of fiber because the body can't fully digest fiber.

A low residue diet restricts foods that contain indigestible material. This causes the body to produce smaller amounts of stool less frequently. A low residue diet is typically recommended for people with inflammatory bowel disease (IBD) flares, for bowel surgery and colonoscopy prep, and for people with infectious colitis or acute diverticulitis.

How does the low residue diet work?

The daily recommended amount of fiber that people should ideally consume is about 25 to 38 grams. However, this may not be right for people with IBD. You should avoid a high fiber diet if you'll be undergoing bowel surgery or if you're experiencing a flare of IBD symptoms.

When following a low residue diet, typical advice is to consume no more than 10 to 15 grams of fiber a day. You should also avoid most dairy products and certain types of carbohydrates. They may provoke abdominal cramping and diarrhea. A healthcare professional or dietitian should supervise you if you decide to follow a low residue diet. Your individual needs will determine the amounts and types of food, as well as how long you follow the diet. Low residue diets are usually only recommended for the short term. These are general guidelines for a low residue diet. They can be changed based on how your body reacts to the diet and what your healthcare team recommends.

Foods to eat on a low residue diet

There are many healthy food options on a low residue diet. It's a good idea to talk with a dietitian before starting this type of diet to determine exactly which foods you should eat and how much of each. Here are some good options they may suggest.

1. Refined carbohydrates
A low residue diet includes refined carbohydrates that are easy to digest, such as:
• white bread, rolls, biscuits
• white pasta
• white rice
• saltine crackers
• refined cereal, like puffed rice or corn flakes
• skinless, cooked potatoes

2. Fruits and vegetables
When it comes to fruits, choose ripened, skinless, seedless, varieties that are raw, canned, or cooked. Good options for a low residue diet include:
• apricots
• bananas
• cantaloupe
• honeydew melon

- nectarines
- papaya
- peaches
- plum
- watermelon

When it comes to vegetable intake, plan to include well-cooked or canned options with no skin or seeds, such as:

- artichoke hearts
- asparagus
- beets
- carrots
- eggplant
- green beans
- mushrooms
- potatoes
- pumpkin
- spinach
- yellow squash

A low residue diet may also include small amounts of certain raw vegetables, including:

- shredded lettuce
- skinless, seedless cucumber

3. Milk and other dairy products

A small amount of smooth milk products may be included in a low residue diet, such as:

- milk
- yogurt
- custard
- ice cream
- cottage cheese
- ricotta cheese

4. Meat and other protein sources
When it comes to meat, choose finely ground, well-cooked, or tender options, like:
• beef
• lamb
• veal
• pork
• ham
You may also eat:
• poultry
• fish
• eggs
• organ meats

5. Sauces and condiments
Safe choices for sauces and condiments include:
• butter
• margarine
• vegetable oil
• plain gravy
• honey
• syrup
• salt
• pepper
• spices
• herbs

6. Snacks, sweets, and desserts
If you feel like snacking or having something sweet, try small portions of plain options like:
• cake
• cookies
• custard

- hard candy
- ice cream
- popsicles
- pretzels
- pudding
- sherbet

7. Drinks

It may be necessary to drink additional fluids to avoid constipation when reducing the volume of your stools with a low residue diet. Stick with plenty of:

- water
- clear broths
- clear fruit juice
- strained vegetable juice

How to make it work for you

Here are a few example meals to try on a low residue diet.
For breakfast:

- scrambled eggs
- pancakes or french toast with butter
- pulp-free juice or decaffeinated coffee with milk and sugar

For lunch:

- baked chicken breast with cooked carrots
- cheeseburger with a seedless bun, onion, lettuce, and ketchup
- turkey or chicken sandwich on French bread

For dinner:

- white rice, steamed vegetables, and baked chicken
- baked potato with the skin removed, butter, and sour cream

• broiled fish, asparagus, and pasta with butter or olive oil

Limitations of the Low Residue Diet

The LRD may be beneficial for symptom management during heightened or acute episodes of increased abdominal pain, infection, or inflammation. However, be aware that this diet is not recommended for all those suffering with inflammatory bowel disease or other chronic conditions. LRD will not decrease inflammation nor will it improve the underlying cause of your condition. Following a LRD for a prolonged period might lead to nutrient deficiencies and other gastrointestinal symptoms (e.g., constipation).

Meal prep tips

Good cooking methods for a low residue diet include:
• steaming
• braising
• poaching
• simmering
• microwaving
Low residue foods should be well cooked. Avoid cooking methods such as roasting, broiling, or grilling, which may make food tough or dry.

Sample Menus

Breakfast

½ cup apple juice ½ cup grits w 1 tsp margarine 1 poached egg 1 slice white toast 1-cup skim milk 1-cup decaf coffee

Breakfast
1-cup corn flake cereal 1-cup skim milk 1 ripe banana 1-cup decaf coffee

Lunch
3 oz roast beef/gravy ½ cup mashed potatoes 1-cup steamed carrots 1 dinner roll 1 slice angel food cake 1-cup fruit punch

Lunch
1-cup chicken noodle soup Sandwich: 3 oz turkey, white bread, 1 tsp mayonnaise 1-cup fruit punch

Dinner
3 oz baked chicken 2/3 cup buttered rice ½ cup green beans ½ cup canned peaches 1-cup iced tea

Dinner
3oz baked pork Mashed potatoes 1 tsp margarine/butter 1-cup waxed beans 1-cup sherbet 1-cup Kool-aid

Foods to avoid on a low residue diet

A dietitian can also help you identify foods you should avoid on a low residue diet. Here are some foods that should typically be avoided:
• legumes, nuts, and seeds
• most raw fruits and vegetables
• popcorn

- unprocessed coconut
- most whole grains, including breads or pastas
- figs, prunes, and berries
- dried fruits
- deli meats
- spicy foods and dressings
- caffeine
- prune juice or juice with pulp
- chocolate
- tough, fibrous meats with gristle

When to start a low residue diet

Certain circumstances and conditions may benefit from a low residue diet. Here are some situations where your healthcare team may recommend it.

1. Crohn's disease
Crohn's disease is an autoimmune disorder that causes inflammation that damages the digestive tract. People with a family history are more likely to develop it. It's unclear why the body attacks its own tissues.

There's currently no cure for Crohn's disease. However, diet changes may help you achieve remission. Some people living with Crohn's disease experience bowel obstructions and narrowing of the ileum, or lower small intestine. A low residue diet may aid in a reduction of symptoms like pain and cramping.

However, research has been inconclusive or contradictory on the diet's effectiveness for inflammatory bowel diseases like Crohn's.

More evidence on if the low residue diet is appropriate and effective for people with Crohn's disease is needed.

2. Ulcerative colitis

A low residue diet may also be helpful for those with ulcerative colitis, though a similar lack of consensus exists here, too.

This IBD causes inflammation and ulcers on the inner lining of the large intestine. The irritation may cause some people to lose their appetite and eat less. This could lead to malnutrition. Special diets can sometimes help. A low residue diet could potentially aid in staying well nourished while recovering from a bowel obstruction or surgery.

In preparation for a colonoscop

The goal of a low residue diet is to limit the size and number of stools. Therefore, it may be prescribed to someone who's about to undergo a colonoscopy.

This procedure is used to detect abnormalities in the large intestine and rectum.

What to keep in mind about a low residue diet

Fruits, vegetables, grains, and legumes supply important antioxidants, phytonutrients, vitamins, minerals, and more.

Normally, you should try to consume a balanced diet, unless your healthcare team tells you otherwise, as the low

residue diet may not provide enough of certain nutrients your body needs to function optimally.
All of these nutrients are essential for good health. Supplements may be necessary to correct deficiencies.

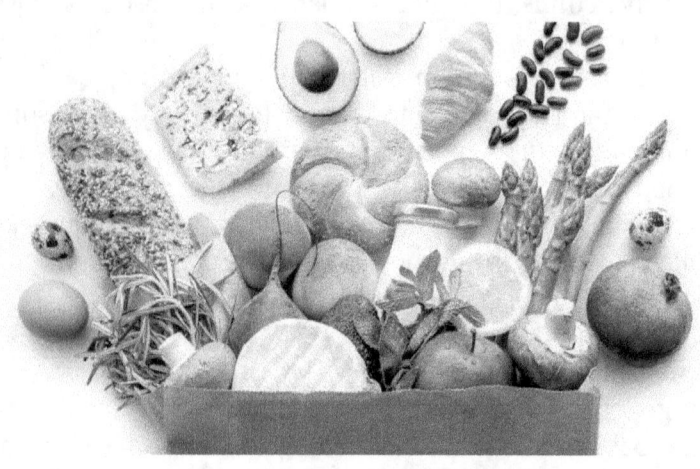

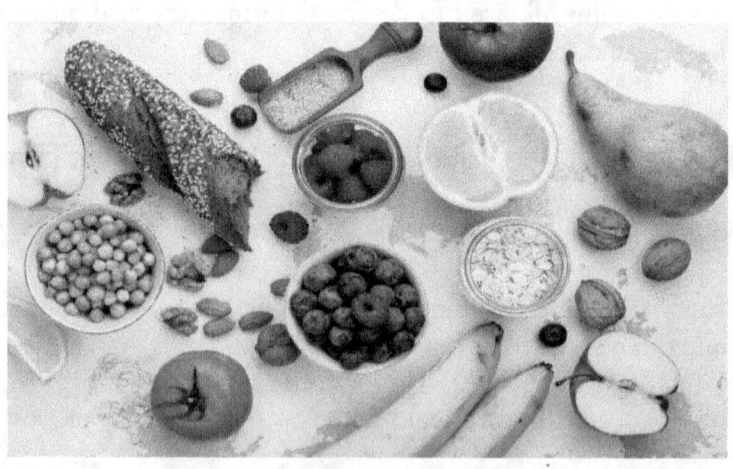

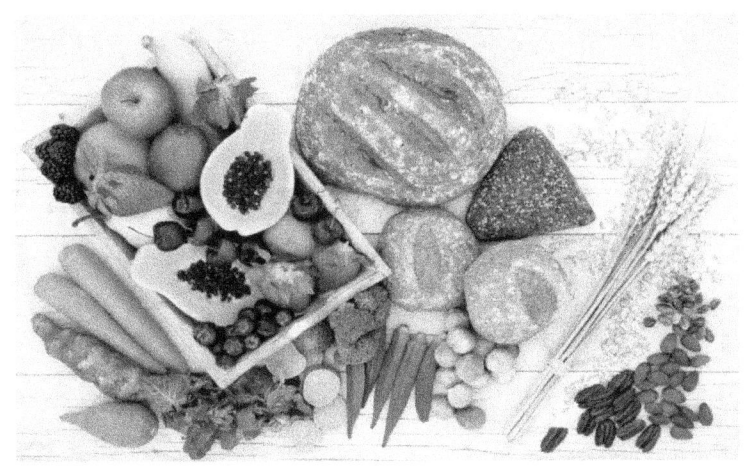

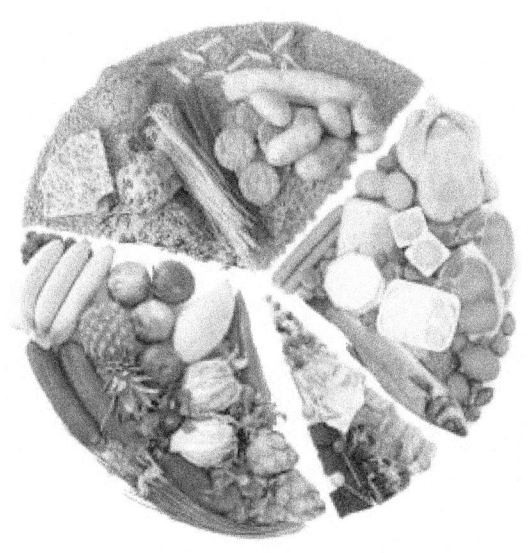

HEALTHY LOW RESIDUE DIET RECIPES

Low Residue Low Fiber Chicken Vegetable Pasta Soup

Ingredients
- 5 cups low sodium chicken broth
- 1 carrot chopped
- 1 potato chopped
- 1/2 cup tomato flesh no skin or seeds
- 1 bunch asparagus tips
- 1/2 cup cooked pastini or other small pasta

Instructions
1. Place broth, carrot and potato in a small saucepan. Bring to a boil, then reduce heat and cook until vegetables are very tender. Add tomatoes and asparagus tips and cook until asparagus is tender. Stir in cooked pasta and cook until heated through.

Low Residue Low Fiber Beet Carrot Soup

Prep Time 5 minutes
Cook Time 30 minutes
Total Time 30 minutes

Ingredients

- 4 cups low sodium vegetable broth
- 1 carrot sliced
- 1 can cooked beets not pickled
- salt to taste
- non-fat yogurt for serving if desired

Instructions

1. Place sliced carrot and vegetable broth in a small saucepan. Bring to a boil, then reduce heat and cook, covered, until carrots are very tender. Add beets and cook until heated through. Pour soup into a blender and puree until smooth. Season to taste with salt. Serve with a spoonful of yogurt stirred in if desired.

Greek Yogurt Fettuccini Alfredo

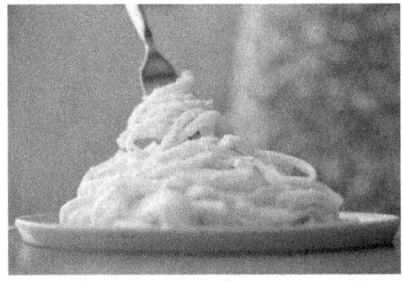

Prep time
10 minutes
Cook Time
15 minutes
Total Time
25 minutes
Yield

Serves 8

Ingredients
1. 1 pound fettuccini
2. 1½ cups whole-milk Greek yogurt
3. ½ cup freshly grated Parmesan, plus more for serving
4. 3 tablespoons minced garlic
5. ¼ cup chopped fresh parsley
6. 1 teaspoon pepper

Instructions
• Boil pasta in salted water per package instructions. Reserve 1 cup cooking liquid, then drain.
• Whisk together yogurt, ½ cup Parmesan, garlic, and parsley. Slowly whisk in cooking liquid a little bit at a time. Add pepper. Pour sauce over pasta and toss to combine.
• Top with more Parmesan to taste and serve immediately. Pasta should register 145 degrees Fahrenheit or higher using an instant-thermometer placed in the middle of the dish.

Super Easy Low Residue Sweet Potato Hash Browns

Ingredients for my super simple Crohn's recipe: sweet potato hash browns
• 2 sweet potatoes
• 1 tbsp gluten-free flour (or the regular kind if you prefer)
• 2 eggs
• 2 tbsp olive oil

Directions for super simple sweet potato hash browns

1. First up, wash and peel sweet potatoes.
2. Use a grater to grate the sweet potatoes in a mixing bowl to create shredded sweet potato.
3. Use a kitchen roll or a cloth to squeeze the sweet potato to get rid of any extra water. This is important to stop them from being soggy or wet when frying!
4. Place your roll/cloth over the mix, press down hard, and squeeze! Keep doing this until the mix is dry and you think you've gotten rid of all the water.
5. Once that's done, break eggs into the bowl and then add a tablespoon of flour.
6. Mix and coat the sweet potatoes well with the egg and flour.
7. In your frying pan, add olive oil and heat.
8. Use your hands to squash your sweet potato into patty-like shapes.
9. Fry each patty for around 5 minutes until golden brown, then serve.

Super Simple Gnocchi and Avocado Bake (Low-Residue)

Ingredients for super simple gnocchi and avocado bake
• 250g of gnocchi (this is usually the size of store-bought gnocchi)
• 1 cup of smooth tomato passata
• 1 avocado mashed
• 1 teaspoon of paprika
• 1/2 teaspoon of turmeric
• A slice of lemon

• A handful of dairy-free grated cheese

Method for super simple gnocchi and avocado bake
1. Boil gnocchi in pan for around 3 minutes; until boiled and gnocchi rises to the top and has softened.
2. Drain the water and pour it out into an oven dish.
3. Stir in the tomato passata and coat gnocchi well.
4. Peel, slice and mash 1 avocado well and stir in with passata and gnocchi.
5. Add turmeric and paprika, coating well.
6. Sprinkle over the dairy-free grated cheese.
7. Cook for 15 minutes, until cheese melts. (The gnocchi is already cooked.)
8. Squeeze over a slice of lemon and serve.

Low-Residue Turmeric Fish With Baked Sweet Potato and Avocado

Ingredients for my low-residue turmeric fish with sweet potato and avocado
• 1 sea bass fillet
• 1 sweet potato
• 1 teaspoon of dairy-free butter
• 1/2 teaspoon of turmeric
• 1/2 teaspoon of cinnamon
• 1 small piece of ginger
• 1 teaspoon of paprika
• 1 teaspoon of olive oil, or any cooking oil of choice (you could also use a low-fat cooking spray)
• 1/2 avocado

- 1/2 lemon
- Optional: 1 spoonful of sauerkraut

Directions for low-residue turmeric fish with sweet potato and avocado
1. Place fish on a baking tray and cover with 1 teaspoon of olive oil or spray with low-fat cooking spray.
2. Peel and chop avocado and place on top of fish.
3. Peel and finely chop the ginger.
4. Mix together in a small bowl: turmeric, paprika, chopped ginger, and cinnamon.
5. Once mixed, spoon over fish and ensure it's evenly coated (the oil/spray will help it stick).
6. Chop and squeeze 1/4 of lemon over the fish.
7. Cook for 20 minutes in the oven at 200 degrees.
8. The sweet potato can be baked in the oven separately – allow 40 minutes in the oven or microwave for 7 minutes.
9. One cooked, serve with a slice of lemon and (optional) sauerkraut.
10. Add the baked sweet potato as a side dish and use dairy-free butter or coconut oil for the sweet potato to soften.

Zucchini Noodles With Ginger-Peanut Sauce

Ingredients
- 3 Tbsp. natural creamy peanut butter
- 2 Tbsp. lower-sodium soy sauce
- 1 ½ tsp. freshly grated ginger
- Juice of 1 lime
- 2 tsp. pure maple syrup

• 2 Tbsp. extra-virgin olive oil, divided
• 1 (14-oz.) block extra-firm tofu, drained, patted dry, and cut into 1-in. cubes
• ½ tsp. kosher salt, divided
• 1 ½ cups matchstick carrots
• 1 red bell pepper, thinly sliced
• 4 medium zucchinis, trimmed and spiralized into thin noodles

Directions
1. In a small bowl, combine peanut butter, soy sauce, ginger, lime juice, and maple syrup, stir with a whisk. Set aside.
2. Heat 1 Tbsp. oil in a large nonstick skillet over medium. Add tofu; cook 8 to 10 minutes or until tofu is golden and crisp, stirring occasionally. Season tofu with ¼ tsp. salt; transfer to a plate.
3. Add remaining 1 Tbsp. oil to pan. Cook carrots and bell pepper until softened, about 5 to 6 minutes, stirring occasionally. Season with remaining ¼ tsp. salt.
4. Add zucchini noodles to pan; cook 2 to 3 minutes, tossing often, to heat through but not fully cook. Add tofu and half of peanut sauce to skillet; gently toss to combine.
5. Divide zucchini noodle mixture evenly between 4 plates. Drizzle remaining peanut sauce over the top.

RAW APPLE CARROT CAKE

Ingredients

1. 2 carrots, grated

2. 2 apples, grated
3. 115g pecans, finely ground
4. 85g desiccated coconut
5. 2tbsp lucuma powder
6. 2tbsp raw cacao powder
7. ½ tsp ground cinnamon
8. Pinch of salt
9. 150g raisins
10. 60g dried apple, soaked for 15 minutes
11. 60g dates, soaked for 15 minutes
12. 1 whole orange, peeled

Instructions

1. Finely grate the apple and carrots. Place in a large bowl with the nuts, lucuma, cacao, cinnamon, salt and raisins.
2. Drain the dried apple and dates and place in a blender with the orange. Process to form a paste. Add to the nut mixture and combined thoroughly. Place the mixture in batches in a food processor and pulse to form a wet dough. Do not over mix.
3. Press the mixture into a greased, lined 20cm (8inch) cake tin and chill for 2-3 hours before serving.

RICE CONGEE

Ingredients

1. 1tbsp olive oil, coconut oil or ghee
2. 2 tablespoons minced ginger optional
3. 1-2 cloves garlic, minced -optional
4. 175g jasmine rice

5. 1600ml vegetable or chicken stock
6. 1 tsp sea salt
7. Tamari soy sauce for flavouring
8. Chopped chives for topping
9. Optional add ins – cooked shittake mushrooms, cooked plain chicken, handful of soaked sea vegetables

Directions
1. Rinse the rice with 2 changes of water. Drain and set aside.
2. Heat the oil in a large saucepan. Once hot, add the ginger and garlic and cook for 30 seconds, until they start to become fragrant. Add the drained rice, and sauté for another minute.
3. Carefully pour the broth. Sprinkle in the salt and stir. Bring the broth to a boil, uncovered. Then, turn the heat to a very low heat and cover. Let it simmer for 1 hour – do not take off the lid.
4. Turn off the heat and leave to sit for 15 minutes.
5. Serve the congee in bowls. Top with a little tamari soy sauce, chopped chives if wished.

Pasta Bake

Ingredients
1. 500 g peeled pumpkin or sweet potato cut into chunks
2. 200 g tinned asparagus cut into chunks
3. 400 g pasta
4. 50 g white bread broken up into crumbs
5. 2 tbsp oil (preferably olive oil)
6. 400 ml vegetable or chicken stock

7. 150 g grated cheese
8. 1 tsp mixed herbs

Directions
1. Preheat the oven to 220C (fan forced)
2. Place the pumpkin/sweet potato in a baking dish and drizzle with one tablespoon of olive oil and roast until the vegetables soft and golden
3. At the same time boil the pasta until al dente and drain
4. In a bowl add breadcrumbs, stock, and the rest of the olive oil, mix until breadcrumbs dissolve then add asparagus, pumpkin, mixed herbs, add pasta and mix 100 grams of the cheese through
5. Place in a baking dish and heat through for 30 minutes finish off with the last 50 grams of cheese on top of the dish for 10 minutes until melted
6. Serve with salad or steamed greens

Spinach & Mushroom Quiche

Ingredients
• 2 tablespoons extra-virgin olive oil
• 8 ounces sliced fresh mixed wild mushrooms such as cremini, shiitake, button and/or oyster mushrooms
• 1 ½ cups thinly sliced sweet onion
• 1 tablespoon thinly sliced garlic
• 5 ounces fresh baby spinach (about 8 cups), coarsely chopped
• 6 large eggs
• ¼ cup whole milk
• ¼ cup half-and-half

- 1 tablespoon Dijon mustard
- 1 tablespoon fresh thyme leaves, plus more for garnish
- ¼ teaspoon salt
- ¼ teaspoon ground pepper
- 1 ½ cups shredded Gruyère cheese

Directions

1. Preheat oven to 375 degrees F. Coat a 9-inch pie pan with cooking spray; set aside.
2. Heat oil in a large nonstick skillet over medium-high heat; swirl to coat the pan. Add mushrooms; cook, stirring occasionally, until browned and tender, about 8 minutes. Add onion and garlic; cook, stirring often, until softened and tender, about 5 minutes. Add spinach; cook, tossing constantly, until wilted, 1 to 2 minutes. Remove from heat.
3. Whisk eggs, milk, half-and-half, mustard, thyme, salt and pepper in a medium bowl. Fold in the mushroom mixture and cheese. Spoon into the prepared pie pan. Bake until set and golden brown, about 30 minutes. Let stand for 10 minutes; slice. Garnish with thyme and serve.

TURMERIC CHICKEN AND SWEET POTATO THAI CURRY

INGREDIENTS
- 2 sweet potatoes
- 2 medium sized potatoes
- 4 chicken breasts
- a handful spinach (to garnish)
- 2 tbsp olive oil

- 1/2 cup coconut milk
- 1/2 cup almond milk
- 1 tbsp chopped ginger
- 3 tbsp of thai green curry paste
- 1 tbsp of turmeric
- 1/4 tbsp of black pepper

INSTRUCTIONS

1. Peel and slice the potatoes and sweet potatoes into small chunks.Place in a pan of cold water and bring to the boil. Then leave to simmer until soft (around 25-30 minutes)

2. In a separate pan, heat olive oil and then add ginger (chopped and diced) and 3 tablespoons of thai green curry paste

3. Add coconut milk and almond milk to the pan gradually, stirring as you go to make a smooth mixture. Cook for 3 minutes to bring out flavours.

4. Dice chicken into small pieces and add to the mixture.

5. Cover chicken in the milk/curry mixture and fry on low heat for 10 minutes

6. Sprinkle over turmeric and black pepper

7. Check the chicken is cooked through (and not pink in the middle). Once cooked it should now be time to add the potato/sweet potato

8. Finally, add potato/sweet potato the pan and coat well with the mixture.

9. Take off heat and sprinkle over fresh, chopped spinach. And enjoy!

Lean Meat and Chicken Stew with Chunky Vegetables (Low-Residue Diet)

Ingredients

Lean Meat and Chicken Stew with Chunky Vegetables
1. 1 tablespoon oil
2. 4 ounces meat
3. 2 chicken thighs
4. 1 onion, diced
5. 4 cloves garlic, minced or 4 cubes Gefen Frozen Garlic
6. 1 sweet potato, peeled and chopped
7. 1 potato, peeled and chopped
8. 2 large carrots, peeled and chopped
9. 3 heaping tablespoons Tuscanini Tomato Paste
10. 8 cups chicken broth (I like to use Manischewitz Low-Sodium and add salt to my preference)
11. 1 teaspoon onion powder
12. salt
13. pepper

Directions
1. Heat the oil until it's screaming hot. Season the meat and chicken with salt and pepper. Add the chicken and meat to the pot and sear for two minutes on each side or until golden on the outside. Remove the chicken and meat to a plate.
2. To the same pot, add the onion, garlic, sweet potato, potato and carrots. Let them sauté until they start getting soft (do not cook them through at this point). Add tomato paste and let it cook for two more minutes. Add the chicken broth, onion powder, and salt and pepper to taste. Bring to a

boil. Reduce the heat and let it simmer for two to four hours. The longer it sits, the better the flavor!

Healthy Low Fat Fried Rice

Ingredients
• Low-fat cooking spray
• 3 eggs plus 2 egg whites lightly beaten
• ground black pepper
• 2 cups long-grain rice cooked and chilled
• 7 water chestnuts sliced
• 1 tablespoon anchovy paste
• 1 tablespoon light soy sauce or more depending on taste
• 1 tablespoon light-dark soy sauce
• 2 spring onions trimmed and sliced into rounds
• 1 cup leftover or cooked chicken or whatever meat you want to use

Instructions
• Heat a non-stick wok until hot and coat with cooking spray.
• Pour in the eggs and scramble, scraping the bits that stick to the wok. Once cooked, remove from the wok and set aside.
• Add a bit more cooking spray to the wok. Add spring onions and anchovy paste and heat through.
• Add the rice, scraping the bottom of the wok and tossing the rice until it's heated through.
• Once the rice is hot, add the remaining ingredients (including the eggs), Continue to cook over medium heat, mixing continuously for 2- 3 minutes.

• Taste and season with pepper and any additional soy sauce that may be needed.

Stir-Fry Velveted Chicken and Vegetables

Ingredients
Velveted Chicken
• 1 pound boneless skinless chicken breast
• 1/2 teaspoon salt
• 1 tablespoon rice wine
• 1 large egg white
• 1 tablespoon cornstarch
• 2 tablespoons oil
Vegetables
• 3 cups chicken broth or water
• 1 carrot peeled, cut into 1/2" thick slices
• 4 shitake mushrooms stems removed, quartered
• 1 medium zucchini peeled, seeds scooped out, sliced into 1/2" thick slices
• 1 bunch asparagus tips
Stir-Fry Sauce
• 1 tablespoon soy sauce
• 1 tablespoon oyster sauce
• 1 tablespoon rice wine
• 1/2 teaspoon sugar
• 2 teaspoons cornstarch dissolved in 2 tablespoons cold water
• 2 teaspoons sesame oil
Stir-Fry
• 2 teaspoons oil
• 1 slice ginger peeled, finely minced

• 1/4 cup low sodium chicken stock

Instructions
Velveting Chicken
1. Cut chicken into thin slices, small cubes, or thin strips. Place in bowl and add salt and rice wine; mix well. Whisk egg white with fork until gel is broken down. Add to chicken, along with cornstarch; mix well. Add 1 tablespoons of oil and stir until well mixed. Cover and refrigerate for at least 30 minutes.
2. Bring 1 quart of water to a boil. Add 1 tablespoon oil and reduce heat to low. Transfer chicken into pot and stir to separate pieces. Continue to stir until coating turns white. Then immediately strain in colander.
Cooking Vegetables
1. Bring chicken broth to a boil in a saucepan. Add carrot slices. Cook until tender. Remove from pan with slotted spoon. Add mushrooms and zucchini to chicken broth and cook until tender. Remove from pan with slotted spoon. Add asparagus tips to pan and cook until tender. Remove from pan with slotted spoon. Reserve 1/4 chicken broth stir-fry; store remaining broth for another use
Sauce
1. In a small bowl, mix together Stir-Fry Sauce ingredients.
Stir-Frying Chicken and Vegetables
1. Heat oil in a wok or large skillet. Add ginger and stir-fry briefly until fragrant. Add cooked vegetables to wok. place velveted chicken on top. Add 1/4 cup chicken stock to wok and cover. Cook on high for 1 minute.
2. Add Stir-Fry Sauce and toss well for 1 minute to coat chicken and vegetables with sauce. Serve

The Creamiest Low-Carb Vegetable Soup

Ingredients (makes 8 servings)
- 700 g cauliflower (1.5 lb)
- 500 g zucchini (1.1 lb)
- 1 clove garlic
- 1 small brown onion (70 g/ 2.5 oz)
- 2 celery stalks (80 g/ 2.8 oz)
- 2 tbsp ghee or butter (30 g/ 1.1 oz)
- 2 cups chicken broth or vegetable stock (480 ml/ 16 fl oz)
- 2 cups water (480 ml/ 16 fl oz)
- 1 tsp fresh thyme, plus extra for garnish
- 1/2 tsp onion powder
- sea salt and pepper to taste
- 1 cup cream (240 ml/ 8 fl oz)
- 4 tbsp extra virgin olive oil (60 ml)

Instructions
1. Wash the vegetables. Remove the green parts of the cauliflower. Peel the onion and garlic.
2. Heat the ghee over medium to high heat in a large saucepan. Chop the onion and garlic finely and sauté until translucent.
3. Add chopped cauliflower, zucchini, celery and seasonings.
4. Add broth and water and bring to the boil. Place a lid on the saucepan and reduce to a simmer. Cook until vegetables are soft, for about 15 minutes.
5. Remove from heat and use an immersion mixer to puree until smooth. Add cream and return to heat until heated through.
6. Serve with a drizzle of olive oil (about 1/2 tablespoon per serving) and a sprig of thyme.

Fruity sponge cake

Ingredients
- butter or oil, for greasing
- 50g plain flour
- 3 tbsp cornflour
- 1 tsp baking powder
- 4 eggs, separated
- 175g caster sugar

For the filling
- 295g can mandarin segment, drained
- 200g tub low-fat fromage frais
- icing sugar, for dusting

Method
- STEP 1: Heat oven to 180C/fan 160C/gas 4. Grease then line the base and sides of 2 x 20cm sandwich tins with greaseproof paper. Sieve the flours and baking powder together.
- STEP 2: Use electric hand beaters to whisk the egg whites until stiff, then briefly whisk in the sugar. Beat the egg yolks quickly, then whisk into the whites. Fold in the dry ingredients using a large metal spoon, then spoon the mixture into the tins and level the tops. Bake for 18-20 mins until risen, light golden and a skewer inserted into the middle comes out clean. Cool in the tins for 10 mins, then gently remove and leave to cool completely.
- STEP 3: Mix the mandarins and fromage frais together. Peel away the greaseproof paper, sandwich the cakes with the mandarin mix, then dust with the icing sugar to serve. Best eaten on the day it's made.

Chicken Breast in White Sauce (Low Fat)

Ingredients
• 4 chicken breasts skinless, whole or cut down the middle
• 2 tablespoons (30 g) butter
• 2¾ tablespoons (25 g) flour
• 1½ cups less 2tbsp (330 ml) semi-skimmed/light milk or half milk half vegetable stock (and omit the stock cube below)
• 4 tablespoons white wine
• 1 teaspoon Dijon mustard
• ½ vegetable stock cube crumbled
• ¼ teaspoon onion granules
• 3 tablespoons fromage blanc/fromage frais or light sour cream
• 2-3 tablespoons olive oil or use cooking spray if you've got a non-stick pan
• pepper to taste plus a little sea salt if needed and fresh herbs for garnish

Instructions
• In a large shallow pan heat 2-3 tablespoons of oil and fry the chicken breasts for 2-3 minutes on each side over a medium heat (or until golden brown). Transfer the chicken onto a plate, cover and set aside (leave the juices, if any, in the pan).
• In the same pan melt the butter over a fairly low heat, add the flour and whisk together until a thick, smooth paste forms (this is roux).
• Add the wine, stir, then add half of the milk, increase the heat and whisk until the sauce starts to thicken. Add the rest of the milk, crumbled stock cube, mustard, onion granules, pepper to taste and continue whisking until the

sauce thickens and starts bubbling up. Whisk in the fromage frais, taste the sauce and adjust the seasoning as necessary.
• Place the chicken back in the pan, coat in the sauce, cover and simmer for 10-15 minutes or until the chicken is fully cooked. Add a splash of water if needed, stir and serve immediately.

Notes
• Cooking times may vary depending on the size of your chicken breasts. If you want to shorten cooking time cut the chicken breasts down the middle before frying. You can also flatten and tenderise the chicken using a meat mallet (or rolling pin) before cooking. This will also shorten cooking time.
• The sauce will thicken after a while so add a splash of water to loosen it (stir it in using a whisk). It is important to use a whisk, rather than a spoon, to make the sauce (to ensure it's smooth).
• Gluten free white sauce: You can replace the wheat flour with corn flour (use 20 g) to make this sauce gluten free.
• Substitutions: Add half the amount of milk and top up with chicken/vegetable stock.
• Seasoning: You may not need to add any salt into the sauce as the stock cube is quite salty. Add plenty of pepper though.
• Best served immediately. Leftovers can be refrigerated, covered, for up to 2 days. Add a splash of water when reheating the sauce (you may have to adjust the seasoning too).

GLUTEN-FREE COCONUT CHICKEN CURRY RECIPE (LOW FODMAP + DAIRY FREE)

INGREDIENTS
FOR THE SPICE BLEND:
• 2 tbsp curry powder (ensure it is low FODMAP - see FAQ section above for links)
• 1 tbsp paprika
• 1 tsp cinnamon
• 1/2 tsp ground ginger
• 1/2 tsp asafoetida
FOR THE CURRY:
• 1 tbsp garlic infused olive oil
• 2 chicken breasts chopped
• 200 ml canned coconut milk 180ml if low FODMAP elimination phase
• 200 ml Greek yoghurt lactose-free if low FODMAP, dairy-free coconut yoghurt if dairy-free
• 1 tbsp tomato puree
• 1 tbsp lemon juice optional
• 1-2 handfuls of spinach
TO SERVE:
• handful of fresh chives chopped
• fresh coriander
• basmati rice I add 1 tsp of turmeric to mine to make it yellow

INSTRUCTIONS
• Place your pan over a medium heat and add a tbsp of garlic-infused oil. Once heated, add your chicken chunks and fry until almost sealed.
• Add your spice mix and stir fry for 1 minute.

• Next add your coconut milk and tomato puree. Stir and then simmer for about 10-15 minutes.
• Add your spinach and lemon juice, if using. Cook until the spinach has wilted down.
• Lastly, add your yoghurt and mix in.
• Sprinkle of some fresh chives and top with fresh coriander! Serve up with basmati rice and my 3-ingredient gluten-free naan bread.

Greek-Style Stuffed Tomatoes

INGREDIENTS
• 8 medium or large heirloom tomatoes or on-the-vine tomatoes
• ¼ cup pine nuts
• 1 cup chopped yellow onion
• 2 cloves garlic, minced
• 1 teaspoon dried oregano
• ¼ teaspoon sea salt
• ⅛ teaspoon freshly ground black pepper
• 1½ cups cooked short grain brown rice
• 1¼ cups coarsely chopped fresh parsley
• 2 tablespoons dried currants

INSTRUCTIONS
1. Preheat oven to 350°F. Cut a thin slice off bottoms of tomatoes so they stand upright. Slice ¼ inch off tops of tomatoes; set tops aside. Using a small spoon or melon baller, scoop out tomato pulp; chop pulp.

2. In a large, dry skillet heat pine nuts over medium 3 to 4 minutes or until golden, stirring occasionally. Remove pine nuts.

3. For stuffing, in the same skillet cook onion in ¼ cup water over medium heat 10 minutes or until translucent. Add tomato pulp, garlic, oregano, salt, and pepper. Cook 5 minutes or until garlic is softened. Stir in rice, parsley, currants, and 3 Tbsp. of the pine nuts. Cook just until rice is heated through. Cool slightly.

4. Fill tomato shells with stuffing. Place in a shallow baking dish; replace tomato tops. Spoon any extra stuffing around tomatoes. Pour enough water into dish to cover bottom. Bake, covered with foil, 30 minutes. Remove foil; bake 10 minutes more.

5. Sprinkle tomatoes with the remaining 1 Tbsp. pine nuts. Serve warm or at room temperature.

LOW FODMAP CARROT AND CORIANDER SOUP

INGREDIENTS
- 1 tablespoon olive oil
- Green tops of 4 spring onions, roughly chopped
- 2 heaped teaspoons ground coriander seeds
- 1 tablespoon tomato purée
- 4 medium carrots (approximately 500g), peeled and diced
- 600ml boiling water
- Salt and pepper to season

....
- For the coriander oil

....
- A small bunch of fresh coriander (cilantro)

- 1-2 tablespoons olive oil
- A pinch of salt and pepper

INSTRUCTIONS
1. Heat the olive oil in a medium pan and gently sauté the spring onion tops for a couple of minutes
2. Add the ground coriander, tomato purée, chopped carrots and any coriander stalks from the bunch of fresh coriander, stir then pour in the boiling water and simmer gently for approximately 15 minutes until the carrots are soft
3. Blend the soup to a smooth purée using a hand blender and season with salt and pepper to taste
4. Meanwhile chop the remaining coriander leaves and use a mortar and pestle to grind the leaves, olive oil, salt and pepper to a thin paste
5. Ladle the soup into bowls and serve with a generous drizzle of coriander oil

GLUTEN-FREE COCONUT CHICKEN CURRY RECIPE (LOW FODMAP + DAIRY FREE)

INGREDIENTS
FOR THE SPICE BLEND:
- 2 tbsp curry powder (ensure it is low FODMAP - see FAQ section above for links)
- 1 tbsp paprika
- 1 tsp cinnamon
- 1/2 tsp ground ginger
- 1/2 tsp asafoetida
FOR THE CURRY:
- 1 tbsp garlic infused olive oil

• 2 chicken breasts chopped
• 200 ml canned coconut milk 180ml if low FODMAP elimination phase
• 200 ml Greek yoghurt lactose-free if low FODMAP, dairy-free coconut yoghurt if dairy-free
• 1 tbsp tomato puree
• 1 tbsp lemon juice optional
• 1-2 handfuls of spinach
TO SERVE:
• handful of fresh chives chopped
• fresh coriander
• basmati rice I add 1 tsp of turmeric to mine to make it yellow
INSTRUCTIONS
• Place your pan over a medium heat and add a tbsp of garlic-infused oil. Once heated, add your chicken chunks and fry until almost sealed.
• Add your spice mix and stir fry for 1 minute.
• Next add your coconut milk and tomato puree. Stir and then simmer for about 10-15 minutes.
• Add your spinach and lemon juice, if using. Cook until the spinach has wilted down.
• Lastly, add your yoghurt and mix in.
• Sprinkle of some fresh chives and top with fresh coriander! Serve up with basmati rice and my 3-ingredient gluten-free naan bread.

Lemon Chicken Rice Soup

Ingredients
• 1 carrot peeled, chopped
• 1 celery stalk peeled, chopped

- 1/4 cup medium grain rice such as sushi rice
- 4 cups low sodium chicken broth
- 1 cup cooked chicken breast shredded
- 3 large eggs
- 1 lemon juiced
- 2 cups baby spinach

Instructions

1. Place carrots, celery, rice and chicken broth in Instant Pot. Cook on high pressure for 10 minutes. Let naturally release 15 minutes; release remaining pressure.
2. Remove cover and set Instant Pot to saute function on high. Stir in chicken. Cook until heated through.
3. Whisk eggs with lemon juice. Gradually whisk a ladle of hot broth into eggs. Whisk eggs into soup pot. Add spinach leaves and stir. Cook until just tender

Roasted Squash and Parmigiano Reggiano Stuffed Pasta

Ingredients
- 1 kg Crown Prince squash or other hard squash, like butternut
- 1 tbsp extra virgin olive oil
- 3 fat garlic cloves skin on
- 6 sage leaves
- 35 g dry breadcrumbs I use panko
- 100 g Parmigiano Reggiano cheese grated
- Zest of one lemon
- 8 sage leaves chopped

- 1/2 tsp nutmeg more if not freshly grated
- 175 g large pasta shells about 2/3 typical box

Marinara sauce
- 2 tsp extra virgin olive oil
- 1 small onion diced
- 2 cloves garlic minced
- 2 tbsp fresh thyme leaves or 1 tsp dried
- 700 g jarred tomatoes chopped
- 1 tsp Balsamic vinegar optional
- salt, pepper and honey to taste

No-cook Parmigiano Reggiano Sauce
- 100 g Parmigiano Reggiano grated
- 3 tbsp créme fraîche
- 1 tbsp milk
- extra grated Parmigiano Reggiano to serve
- chopped parsley to serve

Metric - US Customary

Instructions
- Heat the oven to 180C fan/200C/400F. Cut the squash into about 8 slices, removing the seeds and rubbing the slices and garlic with the oil. Lay on a baking tray, tucking the sage leaves under. Roast in the hot oven for 40 minutes, turning once.
- Scoop the soft squash flesh into a food processor along with the garlic (pop from its skins first), Parmigiano Reggiano, fresh and roasted sage leaves, lemon zest and nutmeg. Blend just until mixed; add the bread crumbs and pulse until mixed - or hand mix them in. Scrape this mixture into a bowl and set aside. May be refrigerated and used within three days at this point.

Marinara sauce

• Heat the oil over a low-medium flame and add the onion, sauting for five minutes, stirring occasionally. Add the garlic and thyme leaves, cooking for a further two minutes. Pour in the tomatoes and their juices and cook for 20 minutes, so that it is just bubbling. Add in balsamic vinegar if using then taste for seasoning, adding salt, pepper and honey/sugar if you wish. I sometimes add a pinch of dried vegetable bouillon. Blend or mash to make it mostly smooth but with some texture. Or leave as chunky.

Pasta

• Cook pasta as directed, drain and rinse with water. Leave to cool a bit.

No-cook Parmigiana Reggiano white sauce

• Mix the ingredients together and set aside. You want a loose, pourable sauce so adjust as needed to achieve this.

Assemble and Bake

• Turn the oven down to 160C fan/180C/350F. To assemble the dish for baking, pour the marinara sauce into a shallow, wide baking dish. Take the cooked pasta shells and spoon the mixture evenly into each one, placing them in the dish as you fill them. Once filled, pour the white sauce over and bake in a oven for 20 minutes, or until the white sauce is lightly browned in patches. Pull from the oven and serve with extra grated Parmigiano Reggiano and chopped parsley

Healthy Fried Rice Recipe

Ingredients

• 1 tablespoon avocado oil (or other healthy cooking oil), divided

- 3 large eggs
- 5–6 scallions (aka green onions), root and 2 inches of green top removed, chopped (about 1/2 cup)
- 1 large carrot, shredded or julienned (about 1/2 cup)
- 1/2 cup frozen peas
- 2 cups cooked brown rice*
- 3 tablespoons organic tamari** or low sodium soy sauce
- 1 teaspoon rice vinegar (no sugar added)
- 1 teaspoon toasted sesame oil
- 1/2 teaspoon freshly grated ginger
- big pinch of sea salt (more or less to taste)
- a few spins freshly ground black pepper

Instructions
1. Heat 1/2 tablespoon oil over medium heat.
2. In a mixing bowl, whisk the eggs into a uniform mixture until well combine and season with a small pinch of sea salt and fresh black pepper.
3. Add the eggs to the pan and scramble. Once cooked remove the scrambled eggs from the pan to a plate and reserve for later.
4. Add the remaining 1/2 tablespoon oil to the pan over medium heat; add the scallions and carrot and sauté 3-4 minutes until softened.
5. Add the frozen peas to the pan, then add the rice, tamari, rice vinegar, toasted sesame oil and ginger. Stir well to combine, the heat from the pan will quickly defrost the peas.
6. Turn off the heat and stir in the scrambled eggs. Season with a pinch of sea salt if needed–it will depend on the sodium content of the tamari and other ingredients.
7. Turn the heat to low and cook another 5 minutes until the entire dish is warmed through.

8. Water chestnuts, bean sprouts, edamame, just about any other veggie you like, or plain shredded chicken would also be a delicious addition to this dish.

Low FODMAP Cottage Pie

Ingredients for low FODMAP cottage pie
• 1 tablespoon onion infused oil
• 1 tablespoon garlic infused oil
• 1 large carrot peeled and chopped
• 1 medium zucchini, chopped
• 1 celery stalk, chopped (this small quantity of celery per serving is low FODMAP)
• ½ teaspoon dried thyme
• 2 lbs lean ground beef
• 4 tablespoons low FODMAP gravy powder (make sure the ingredients are low FODMAP)
• 1 cup beef or vegetable stock
• 1 large can chopped tomatoes
• salt and pepper to taste
• 2 cups cheddar cheese, grated

Ingredients for the mashed potato
• 1 tablespoon salt
• 2.2 pounds or about 12 medium size potatoes that are most suitable for mashing, peeled and quartered in even size
• 8 tablespoons butter, softened but not melted (or non-dairy alternative)
• 1 cup lactose free milk, warm to hot (or other low FODMAP non dairy alternatives like rice milk, almond/coconut milk etc.)

Directions for low FODMAP cottage pie
1. Heat the onion and garlic infused oils in a large non sticky pan.
2. Stir fry the chopped carrot, zucchini and celery stalk for a few minutes until softened.
3. Add the minced beef and stir with a wooden spoon to break up any lumps.
4. Cook until the meat is browned.
5. Add gravy powder and stir well.
6. Add stock liquid and stir well.
7. Add canned chopped tomato.
8. Add thyme.
9. Add salt and pepper to taste.
10. Stir well and simmer on low-medium heat for about 30 minutes or until thickened, stirring regularly.
11. Spoon meat into a large casserole dish.
12. Sprinkle half the cheese on the meat.
13. Using a pipe or just a spoon cover evenly with mashed potatoes.
14. Sprinkle the other half of the cheese on the potatoes.
15. Preheat oven to 390 F fan-forced and cook for around 30 mins, or until the mashed potato topping is of a lovely golden brown colour.

Directions for the mashed potato
1. While the meat is cooking, start the mashed potatoes.
2. Peel the potatoes and rinse them under cold water.
3. In a large saucepan, cover the potatoes with cold water, add salt in the water and bring to the boil.
4. Turn the heat down and simmer until tender (after approximately 12 minutes insert a knife in one of the potatoes to see if it's cooked all the way through).
5. Drain well and mash immediately using a masher.

6. Incorporate the butter, using a spoon and stir vigorously.

7. Slowly add the hot milk until the right consistency is reached.

8. Add salt to taste and set aside for a minute while you put the cooked meat onto a casserole dish.

Roasted asparagus

INGREDIENTS
• 500 g asparagus
• 2 tablespoon olive oil
• good pinch salt and pepper
• fresh lemon for squeezing – optional

INSTRUCTIONS
• Preheat the oven to 200°C (400°F).
• Snap the woody ends off the asparagus and discard. Wash the spears well.
• Spread the asparagus out on a large baking tray. Drizzle over the oil and season with the salt and pepper. Use your hands to toss the asparagus in the oil until they are coated, then spread out in a single layer.
• Roast the asparagus at 200°C (400°F) until cooked and just beginning to char. This will be approx. 8-10 minutes for thin spears, 10-12 minutes for thicker asparagus.
• Pile onto a serving dish, squeeze over some fresh lemon juice if you're using it, and eat hot!

Low fodmap pasta sauce

INGREDIENTS
• 1 (28-ounce) can whole peeled tomatoes
• ¼ cup garlic-infused olive oil
• 1 teaspoon dried basil
• ½ teaspoon dried oregano
• ⅛ teaspoon red pepper flakes, optional
• Salt and pepper

INSTRUCTIONS
1. Place tomatoes, olive oil, basil, oregano, and optional red pepper flakes in a blender. Pulse until your desired sauce consistency is achieved.
2. Pour sauce into a large saucepan and heat over medium-high heat. Bring to a boil. Reduce heat to medium-low and simmer, stirring occasionally, for 10 minutes. Season with salt and pepper. Add more basil, oregano, or red pepper flakes, if desired.
3. Serve warm over your favorite low FODMAP pasta.

NOTES
1. Whole Peeled Tomatoes: A low FODMAP serving is a ½ cup or 92 grams. This pasta sauce makes about 8 servings, which works out to be ~99 grams of canned tomatoes. Although this is a slightly larger amount than recommended for a green serve, it may be tolerated. If you'd like to be safe, divide this sauce into 9 or 10 servings instead.

Garlic and onion-free taco seasoning

INGREDIENTS
- 2 tablespoons ground ancho chili pepper
- 2 teaspoons ground cumin
- 2 teaspoons ground paprika
- 1 teaspoon ground oregano
- 1 teaspoon salt
- ½ teaspoon ground cayenne pepper

INSTRUCTIONS
1. Mix together ground chili pepper, cumin, paprika, oregano, salt, and cayenne pepper.
2. Store in an airtight container at room temperature until ready to use.

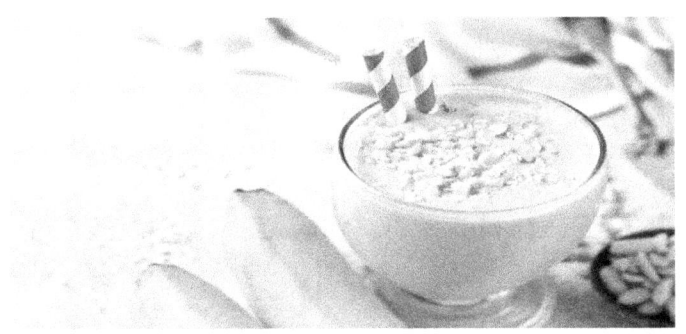

HEALTHY SMOOTHIE RECIPE

Protein Smoothie recipes for Low residue diet

GUT FRIENDLY SMOOTHIE

INGREDIENTS
- 1 banana
- 1 tablespoon of cashew nut butter
- 1 tablespoon of ground turmeric and sprinkle of black pepper
- 2 thumb size pieces of ginger, chopped finely and peeled
- I added these extra ingredients but these are optional depending on how you tolerate them. Although the seeds might like really tough, once they're blended in the smoothie, you should do just fine (especially with Chai since it's mainly soluble fibre. If you are cautious, then please try them one at a time.
- 1 teaspoon of Chia seeds
- 1 teaspoon of Hemp Powder
- 1/4 cup of gluten-free Muesli or oats, I used Delicious Alchemy's Gluten Free Muesli
- 1 cup of Almond Milk, I use Alpro Unsweetened because it's one of the few that are carrageenan free- but Rude Health is also a good shout

INSTRUCTIONS
1. Whizz all together in the Nutribullet for 30 seconds and voila....the perfect breakfast smoothie.

Green Smoothie Recipe

Ingredients
- 200g baby spinach
- 1 banana
- 1 mango
- 150g plain yoghurt
- 100ml milk
- 1tbsp honey

Method
1. Peel the banana and the mango then cut both of them into small chunks.
2. Put all the ingredients into the jug of a blender, then blend for a couple of minutes or until smooth.
3. Keep in the fridge for a few hours.

Fruit & Yogurt Smoothie

Ingredients
- 3/4 cup nonfat plain yogurt
- 1/2 cup 100% pure fruit juice
- 1 1/2 cups (6 1/2 ounces) frozen fruit, such as blueberries, raspberries, pineapple or peaches

Directions
1. Puree yogurt with juice in a blender until smooth. With the motor running, add fruit through the hole in the lid and continue to puree until smooth.

Low-Calorie Banana & Vanilla Smoothie Recipe

Ingredients
• 250 ml skimmed milk
• 1 small banana, peeled and sliced into chunks
• 2 tbsp fat-free natural yoghurt
• 1 tbsp honey

Method
• Peel and slice the banana into small ½ inch rounds.
• Add the sliced banana along with the milk, yoghurt and honey into a food processor.
• Blend the ingredients on high until you have a smooth consistency.
• If the smoothie is too thick to drink, add a small amount of cold water to loosen the mixture and blend again.
• Pour the smoothie mixture into two glasses and serve immediately.

Jugo Verde (Mexican Green Juice)

EQUIPMENT
• Knife
• Cutting Board
• Blender
• Piitcher or carafe
• Juice glasses

INGREDIENTS
• 2 cups freshly squeezed orange juice chilled

- 4 dinosaur kale leaves
- 1 celery stalk
- 1 pineapple spear
- 1/2 green apple
- 1/3 cucumber with skin
- 10 parsley sprigs

INSTRUCTIONS
- Blend orange juice, fruits, and vegetables until completely smooth.
- Serve chilled.

The Best High Fiber Smoothie (Easy + Healthy!)

INGREDIENTS
- 1 cup frozen mixed berries
- 3/4 cup vanilla Greek yogurt
- 1/2 banana
- 1 tbsp chia seeds
- 1/4 cup oats
- 1 cup almond milk
- 1 tsp honey optional

INSTRUCTIONS
- Add all ingredients to a blender and blend on high for 20-30 seconds

Stir-Fry Velveted Chicken and Vegetables

Ingredients
Velveted Chicken
• 1 pound boneless skinless chicken breast
• 1/2 teaspoon salt
• 1 tablespoon rice wine
• 1 large egg white
• 1 tablespoon cornstarch
• 2 tablespoons oil
Vegetables
• 3 cups chicken broth or water
• 1 carrot peeled, cut into 1/2" thick slices
• 4 shitake mushrooms stems removed, quartered
• 1 medium zucchini peeled, seeds scooped out, sliced into 1/2" thick slices
• 1 bunch asparagus tips
Stir-Fry Sauce
• 1 tablespoon soy sauce
• 1 tablespoon oyster sauce
• 1 tablespoon rice wine
• 1/2 teaspoon sugar
• 2 teaspoons cornstarch dissolved in 2 tablespoons cold water
• 2 teaspoons sesame oil
Stir-Fry
• 2 teaspoons oil
• 1 slice ginger peeled, finely minced
• 1/4 cup low sodium chicken stock

Instructions
Velveting Chicken

1. Cut chicken into thin slices, small cubes, or thin strips. Place in bowl and add salt and rice wine; mix well. Whisk egg white with fork until gel is broken down. Add to chicken, along with cornstarch; mix well. Add 1 tablespoons of oil and stir until well mixed. Cover and refrigerate for at least 30 minutes.

2. Bring 1 quart of water to a boil. Add 1 tablespoon oil and reduce heat to low. Transfer chicken into pot and stir to separate pieces. Continue to stir until coating turns white. Then immediately strain in colander.

Cooking Vegetables

1. Bring chicken broth to a boil in a saucepan. Add carrot slices. Cook until tender. Remove from pan with slotted spoon. Add mushrooms and zucchini to chicken broth and cook until tender. Remove from pan with slotted spoon. Add asparagus tips to pan and cook until tender. Remove from pan with slotted spoon. Reserve 1/4 chicken broth stir-fry; store remaining broth for another use

Stir-Fry Sauce

1. In a small bowl, mix together Stir-Fry Sauce ingredients.

Stir-Frying Chicken and Vegetables

1. Heat oil in a wok or large skillet. Add ginger and stir-fry briefly until fragrant. Add cooked vegetables to wok. place velveted chicken on top. Add 1/4 cup chicken stock to wok and cover. Cook on high for 1 minute.

2. Add Stir-Fry Sauce and toss well for 1 minute to coat chicken and vegetables with sauce. Serve

Raspberry and banana smoothie

Ingredients

- 80g / 3 oz. of fresh or frozen raspberries
- 1 medium banana
- 62g / 2 oz. of low-fat natural yogurt
- 90ml / 3 fl oz. of semi-skimmed milk
- 4 ice cubes
- 90ml / 3 fl oz. of unsweetened orange juice

Methods
1. If using frozen raspberries, boil them for 1 minute.
2. If using fresh raspberries wash them under a running cold tap
3. Peel the banana
4. Make sure all the ingredients are chilled before use
5. Blend fruit, yoghurt, milk and juice together using a hand held blender or a smoothie maker until creamy
6. Add ice cubes and blend again
7. Pour into two glasses and serve immediately

What you will need
- Chopping board
- Chopping knife
- Hand blender

Banana, oat and blueberry breakfast smoothie

Ingredients
- 1/2 cup traditional rolled oats
- 2 ripe bananas
- 1/2 cup frozen blueberries
- 2 tsp LSA (see note)
- 1 cup reduced-fat milk

- 1 cup reduced-fat plain Greek-style yoghurt
- 2 tsp honey

Methods

1. Blend oats, banana, blueberries, LSA, milk, yoghurt and honey together until smooth. Pour into chilled glasses. Serve.

The Best High Fiber Smoothie (Easy + Healthy!)

INGREDIENTS
- 1 cup frozen mixed berries
- 3/4 cup vanilla Greek yogurt
- 1/2 banana
- 1 tbsp chia seeds
- 1/4 cup oats
- 1 cup almond milk
- 1 tsp honey optional

INSTRUCTIONS
- Add all ingredients to a blender and blend on high for 20-30 seconds.

Low Residue Low Fiber Chicken Vegetable Pasta Soup

Ingredients
- 5 cups low sodium chicken broth
- 1 carrot chopped
- 1 potato chopped
- 1/2 cup tomato flesh no skin or seeds
- 1 bunch asparagus tips
- 1/2 cup cooked pastini or other small pasta

Instructions
1. Place broth, carrot and potato in a small saucepan. Bring to a boil, then reduce heat and cook until vegetables are very tender. Add tomatoes and asparagus tips and cook until asparagus is tender. Stir in cooked pasta and cook until heated through.

Two-minute breakfast smoothie

Ingredients
- 1 banana
- 1 tbsp porridge oats
- 80g soft fruit (whatever you have – strawberries, blueberries, and mango all work well)
- 150ml milk
- 1 tsp honey
- 1 tsp vanilla extract

Method
• STEP 1Put all the ingredients in a blender and whizz for 1 min until smooth.
• STEP 2Pour the banana oat smoothie into two glasses to serve.

GUT FRIENDLY GLUTEN FREE PAD THAI

INGREDIENTS
• - 2 cups of rice noodles (pre-cooked or dry depending on preference)
• - 2 chicken breasts, diced
• - 1 courgette
• - 1 tablespoon of coconut oil, or olive oil if preferred
• - 1-2 tablespoons of chicken seasoning
• - 2 tablespoons of gluten-free soy sauce.
• - 1 thumbsize piece of ginger.
• - 1 garlic clove.
• - 1-2 slices of lime
• - 1 teaspoon of cashew nut butter
• -Nutritonal Yeast, optional
• - 1 teaspoon of turmeric, optional
• - Black pepper for seasoning, optional

INSTRUCTIONS
1. Add 2 tablespoons of coconut oil to frying pan and heat.
2. Finely chop ginger and garlic and add to pan. Cook until they brown.
3. Peel and finely slice courgette and add this to the pan.

4. Add diced chicken, and chicken seasoning. cook until lightly browned (around 6-8 minutes)

5. Add in noodles (if you buy dry rice noodles; you'll need to boil these in water beforehand for five minutes) and stir fry with chicken and courgette for 2 minutes.

6. Add soy sauce, turmeric and squeeze over the juice of 1 slice of lime.

7. Add 1 teaspoon of nut butter and melt in pan, stirring through.

8. Turn pan off heat. Add in a sprinkle of black pepper, nutritional yeast and a final squeeze of lime.

Low-FODMAP Peanut & Banana Smoothie

Ingredients
• 1 & 1/2 cups low-FODMAP milk (almond for vegan version or lactose-free 2% milk are my favorites)
• 1 tablespoon peanut butter
• 1 tsp cinnamon
• 1 tablespoon sugar (may also substitute sucralose or stevia)
• 1/3 medium-sized ripe frozen banana (note: banana FODMAP content increases with ripeness. If you select unripe banana for your smoothie you can safely consume up to 1 medium banana)
• 1/2 cup ice cubes

Directions
1. Blend all ingredients on high for 1 minute. Serves 1-2.

Low-FODMAP Wild Blueberry & Chia Smoothie

Ingredients
- 1 & 1/2 cups low-FODMAP milk (I used almond)
- 1/3 cup (28g) wild blueberries (I used fresh frozen)
- since wild blueberries are smaller it is better to weigh than count these
- can also substitute regular blueberries
- 40g is one low-FODMAP serving
- 1 tablespoon chia seeds
- Hint: can also use low-FODMAP chia pudding- just leave seeds in small amount low-FODMAP milk of your choice overnight in refrigerator, the seeds swell and it turns into a nice pudding; here is a great low-FODMAP Chia Pudding recipe
- 1 tablespoon sugar (may also substitute sucralose or stevia)
- 1 tablespoon protein powder (I used Nutribiotic vanilla flavored brown rice protein powder- see the low-FODMAP Travel 10 tip blog for a photo)
- 1/2 cup ice cubes

Direction
1. Blend all ingredients on high for 1 minute. Serves 1-2.

Low-FODMAP Strawberry, Almond & Flax Smoothie

Ingredients
- 1 & 1/2 cups low-FODMAP milk (I used unsweetened almond milk, this is vegan)
- 1 cup (130g; maximum serving is 65 g) fresh frozen strawberries

• 1 tablespoon flax seed meal
• 1 tablespoon almond butter
• 1 tablespoon sugar (may also substitute sucralose or stevia)
• 1/2 cup ice cubes

Directions
1. Blend all ingredients on high for 1 minute. Serves 2.

Oatmeal Smoothie

Ingredients
• 1/4 cup old-fashioned oats or quick oats
• 1 banana chopped into chunks and frozen
• 1/2 cup unsweetened almond milk
• 1 tablespoon creamy peanut butter
• 1/2 tablespoon pure maple syrup plus additional to taste
• 1/2 teaspoon pure vanilla extract
• 1/2 teaspoon ground cinnamon
• 1/8 teaspoon kosher salt don't skip this, as it makes the oatmeal pop!
• Ice optional, add at the end if you want a thicker smoothie

Instructions
• Place the oats in the bottom of a blender and pulse a few times until finely ground. Add the banana, milk, peanut butter, maple syrup, vanilla, cinnamon, and salt.
• Blend until smooth and creamy, stopping to scrape down the blender as needed. Taste and add additional sweetener if you'd like a sweeter smoothie. Enjoy immediately.

Notes
• This smoothie tastes best the day it is made, but can be refrigerated for up to 1 day.
• For fast prep, pre-portion the oats, banana, and spices in a ziptop bag and freeze until needed. Add with the remaining ingredients to a blender and enjoy!

High Fiber Protein Smoothie

INGREDIENTS
• 1 cup unsweetened almond milk or milk of choice
• 1/2 cup frozen strawberries or fruit of choice
• 1/3 cup protein powder
• 1/2 cup white beans drained and rinsed
• 1/2 cup cauliflower rice frozen
• 1 cup spinach
• 1/2 tablespoon ground flax
• Stevia to taste optional

INSTRUCTIONS
• Place all the ingredients into a high-speed blender. Blend until smooth and serve!
• To make your protein smoothie ahead of time, you have two options. First, you can measure the ingredients and place in a food storage bag in the freezer. Then blend when you're ready to eat. Second, you can blend everything together and store in a mason jar or protein shaker in the freezer up to 5 days.

Oats Smoothie for Weight Loss

Ingredients
• 1 whole banana optional: cut into smaller chunks and frozen
• ½ cup rolled oats (or quick oats are okay if that's what you have)
• ½ cup almond milk or oat milk, unsweetened, homemade and organic, OR: Three Trees or Malk brands preferred; if you can, try to avoid all nut and oat milks with added oils and vitamins. Find the above milks in the refrigerator section of many stores.
• ½ cup water
• ⅛ teaspoon sea salt or Potassium Lite Salt

Ingredients
• 1 whole banana optional: cut into smaller chunks and frozen
• ½ cup rolled oats (or quick oats are okay if that's what you have)
• ½ cup almond milk or oat milk, unsweetened, homemade and organic, OR: Three Trees or Malk brands preferred; if you can, try to avoid all nut and oat milks with added oils and vitamins. Find the above milks in the refrigerator section of many stores.
• ½ cup water
• ⅛ teaspoon sea salt or Potassium Lite Salt

Instructions
• Add oats to blender.
• Blend or pulse until mostly powdered or finely ground.
• Add banana. (If frozen, be sure it's cut into smaller chunks or slices.) Top with milk, water and sea salt.

• Blend until smooth and creamy. Enjoy!

Acid Reflux Smoothie

INGREDIENTS
• ¾ cup cashew milk
• 5 fresh basil just leaves
• ¼ cup spinach
• ½ inch ginger root
• 1 banana frozen
• ½ pear
• ⅓ cup rolled oats

INSTRUCTIONS
• Blend cashew milk, basil leaves, and spinach until smooth
• Add remaining ingredients and blend again
• Serve over ice for a refreshingly cool smoothie

NOTES
• Use at least 1 frozen fruit for a cold smoothie.
• Feel free to add more basil or ginger for a bolder flavor

Green Breakfast Smoothie Recipe

Ingredients
• 2 cups spinach or kale leaves (see notes)
• 2 cups chopped pineapple
• 1 medium banana

- ½ apple (chopped)
- 2 tablespoons hemp hearts (sub flax seeds or chia seeds)
- 1-2 cups water (see notes)

Instructions
- Put spinach or kale, pineapple, banana, apple hemp hearts, and 1 cup of the water into a high-powered blender. 2 cups spinach or kale leaves, 2 cups chopped pineapple, 1 medium banana, ½ apple, 2 tablespoons hemp hearts, 1-2 cups water
- Blend for 1 minute until very smooth. If you'd like a thinner smoothie, add more water.
- Pour your breakfast smoothie into a glass and enjoy it right away.

Notes
1. If you don't have a high-powered blender, you can still make this smoothie, but keep in mind that it won't be as smooth. It will still taste delicious!
2. If you're unsure about how a green breakfast smoothie will taste, opt for spinach as it's less green-tasting.
3. Make sure that at least one of the ingredients is frozen. We normally keep a bag of peeled bananas in the freezer for smoothies. If all of your ingredients are fresh, you can add some ice cubes to chill the smoothie.
4. The exact amount of water you need will depend on the size of the banana and apple you use, how many ingredients are frozen, and personal preference. It is best to start with 1 cup and then add more as needed.

CONCLUSION

Your physician or dietitian can help you decide if this diet is right for you and the appropriate length of time for you to follow it. When transitioning from a LRD to your regular diet, be sure to increase fibre gradually, by about 5 grams weekly, until you have reached your fibre goal. It is also important to drink plenty of liquids when increasing dietary fibre.

www.ingramcontent.com/pod-product-compliance
Lightning Source LLC
Chambersburg PA
CBHW062250290526
45794CB00006B/2482